Dental Revision

Questions and Answers
to Pass Exams in Dentistry

M. Assadpour

A CIP catalogue record for this book is available from the British Library.

Library of Congress Control Number: 2016914658

Published by CreateSpace Independent Publishing Platform, North Charleston, South Carolina

ISBN-13: 978-1534874572

ISBN-10: 1534874577

Cover Design: E. Honary

Contents

About This Book

In dental school I was well known for my note taking abilities and revision skills. My extensive and organised collection of revision notes was the subject of envy among my classmates. After graduating as a dentist, I used these same notes to pass my MJDF (Diploma of Membership of the Joint Dental Faculties) exam. A revised version of these notes have now been collected in this book to help you prepare for and pass your dental exams.

Whether you are taking MCQs, writing short essays or preparing for an OSCE, the questions forming this collection are some of the most popular exam questions. The answers are concise but informative. The aim of this book is to help you prepare for a variety of dentistry exams.

The information in this book has come from several sources such as dental textbooks, university lectures, and academic journals. A list of references can be found at the end of the book.

1 Periodontics: Questions

1. What is Necrotising Ulcerative Gingivitis (NUG) and how does it differ from Necrotising Ulcerative Periodontitis (NUP)?

2. What factors contribute to NUG and what are some of its signs and symptoms?

3. Explain how furcation involvement is classified and what probe is used in furcation assessment?

4. What group of people are more likely to be affected by Localised Aggressive Periodontitis?

5. Which area of the mouth is often affected by Localised Aggressive Periodontitis?

6. What is the microorganism most commonly responsible for Localised Aggressive Periodontitis?

7. Name three advantages and three disadvantages of using Locally Delivered Antibiotics (LDA) in treatment of periodontitis.

8. Name two LDA used in treatment of periodontitis.

9. How would you describe a periodontal pocket?

10. What is Biological Width?

11. What is the aim of Non-surgical Periodontal Therapy?

12. What probes can be used in Basic Periodontal Examination (BPE)?

13. Describe a WHO probe.

14. In BPE, what does code 2 signifies? What is the indicated treatment for this code?

15. Why can't BPE be used to assess the effectiveness of periodontal treatment?

16. What does the symbol (*) means in Basic Periodontal Examination?

17. Describe the Silness and Löe Plaque Index.

18. Name two genetic conditions and two systemic diseases that increase the risk of periodontitis.

19. Name three local pre-disposing factors that lead to periodontitis.

20. What is Desquamative gingivitis?

21. Name two drugs that can cause gingival hyperplasia.

22. Name three ways in which smoking contributes to periodontitis.

23. How are the horizontal bitewings useful in periodontal examination?

24. Describe the Miller's classification of tooth mobility.

25. Describes two ways in which Chlorhexidine gluconate mouth rinse is effective in treatment of periodontitis.

2 Periodontics: Answers

1. NUG is the ulceration and necrosis of interdental papillae which can lead to the loss of papillae. NUP can follow NUG and involves more severe attachment loss and vertical bone loss.

2. Factors contributing to NUG are:

   - Smoking
   - Poor oral hygiene
   - Stress
   - Immuno-depression

   Signs and symptoms of NUG:

   - Punched out and ulcerated interdental papillae
   - Halitosis
   - Pain

3. Furcation classifications:

Class I: Tissue destruction doesn't extend more than 1/3 of the tooth width.

Class II: Tissue destruction extends to more than 1/3 of the tooth width.

Class III: Tissue destruction extended the entire width of the tooth.

Naber's probe

4. Children under the age of 14

5. First molars +/- central incisors often in one quadrant of the mouth

6. *Actinobacillus actinomycetemcomitans*

7. Advantages of LDA are:

- Drug delivered in high concentration to the site
- Reduced risk of systemic side effects
- Reduced reliance on patient's compliance

Disadvantages of LDA are:

- Patient misconception

- Time consuming
- Storage requirement

8. Minocycline 2% (Dentocycline), Metronidazole 25% (Elyzol)

9. Periodontal pocket is a sack bound by soft and hard tissue. The soft tissue walls are lined with ulcerated epithelium over an inflamed cementum tissue. The hard tissue wall is the root surface, covered with biofilm which contains bacteria.

10. Biological Width is the combined length of junctional epithelium and connective tissue attachment.

11. The aim of Non-surgical Periodontal Therapy is reattachment of long junctional epithelium to a cleaned root surface

12. WHO/ CPITN probes

13. A WHO (World Health organisation) probe has a 0.5 mm ball-tipped end and a colour coded mark 3.5 mm to 5.5 mm from the tip.

14. Code 2 means there are no pockets larger than 3.5 mm present, there is supra +/-

subgingival calculus present, restoration overhangs present. The treatment includes oral hygiene instructions and removal of plaque retentive factors including calculus

15. Because it doesn't provide information about individual teeth within each sextant. 6 Point Pocket Chart (6 sites per tooth) provides more information.

16. The symbol (*) indicates presence of a furcation

17. In Silness and Löe Plaque Index system, four surfaces of each tooth are examined for the presence of plaque and the findings are scored in the following way:

0:   No plaque present

1:   Film of plaque detected on the surface of the tooth with the help of disclosing agent or a probe

2:   Moderate accumulation of the plaque on the tooth surface visible to naked eye

3:   Abundance of plaque on the surface of the tooth or in the pockets

The total of the scores for all surfaces is divided by the number of surfaces scored.

18. Genetic conditions increasing risk of periodontitis:

- Down's syndrome
- Papillion- Lefevre syndrome

Systemic diseases increasing risk of periodontitis:

- Diabetes Mellitus
- Crohn's disease

19. Poor oral hygiene, smoking

20. Desquamative gingivitis is a diffused erythematous lesion affecting the width of keratinised gingiva. Desquamative gingivitis can be a symptom of a number of conditions such as Lichen planus, Pemphigus vulgaris, Lupus erythematous and pemphigoid.

21. Phenytoin, Cyclosporine

22. Reduced blood flow to the soft tissues, impaired white cell function, increased production of cytokines

23. Subgingival calculus and localised areas of bone loss can be detected on horizontal bite wings.

24. Miller's classification:

Class I: Tooth can be moved less than 1 mm in either buccolingual or mesiodistal directions.

Class II: Tooth can be moved 1 mm or more in buccolingual or mesiodistal directions. There is no vertical mobility.

Class III: Tooth can be moved 1 mm or more in buccolingual or mesiodistal directions and there is vertical mobility.

25. Chlorhexidine gluconate is an antimicrobial agent which increases cellular membrane permeability and reduces the adherence of *prophyromonas gingivalis* to epithelial cells.

3 Endodontics: Questions

1. Explain the difference between reversible pulpitis and irreversible pulpitis.

2. What is Acute Apical Periodontitis?

3. Describe the immediate management of a sodium hypochlorite extrusion injury.

4. Name four reasons for mechanical preparation of root canals.

5. What is EDTA and why is it used in endodontic treatment?

6. Name four types of endodontic sealers.

7. Name two indications and two contra indications for apicectomy.

8. What are three advantages of Crown-Down technique in endodontic?

9. Name 4 ways to prevent instrument fracture (separation) during endodontic treatment.

10. What do we mean by "agitating the irrigants" in endodontic and how can it be done?

11. Name four factors that could improve the outcome of endodontic treatment.

12. What do we mean by the term "Zip and elbow" in endodontic?

13. What is "Apical Gauging" and why is it important?

14. Why is "Glide Path" important in endodontics?

15. Name four ideal properties of a root canal filling material.

16. What are the two aims of obturation in endodontics?

17. Explain the difference between internal root resorption and external root resorption.

18. Name three indications for the use of systemic antibiotics in endodontics.

19. Name four techniques for removal of separated endodontic instruments from the root canal.

20. Name three properties of calcium hydroxide used as endodontic medicament.

21. Explain the difference between Reparative dentine and Reactionary dentine.

22. Explain the differences between a periapical granuloma and a periapical cyst.

23. Name three anatomical landmarks that can be mistaken as periapical lesions when interpreting radiographs.

24. What is Ankylosis?

25. Name four common causes for the persistence or reoccurrence of periapical disease.

26. Explain three advantages of using rubber dam during endodontics.

27. What is a pulp polyp?

28. Describe two clinical situations where pulp testing may be indicated.

29. How does an Electric Pulp Tester (EPT) function?

30. What is Mineral Trioxide Aggregate (MTA) and how is it used in endodontics?

4 Endodontics: Answers

1. Reversible pulpitis:

   - Transient pain in response to temperature stimuli which lasts for a few seconds
   - Pain does not affect sleep
   - No spontaneous pain

   Irreversible pulpitis:

   - Long lasting pain (minutes to hours) in response to temperature stimuli
   - Spontaneous pain
   - Pain disrupts patient's sleep

2. Acute Apical Periodontitis is the inflammation of the apical periodontium caused by occlusal trauma, egress of bacteria from infected pulp, toxins from necrotic pulp or iatrogenic damage caused during endodontic therapy. The tooth is often tender to biting and

widening of periodontal ligament space (PDL) may be seen on the radiograph.

3. Steps in immediate management of a sodium hypochlorite extrusion injury:
    -   Irrigate the canals with water or saline and leave open to drain.
    -   Periapical radiograph to identify the cause of extrusion.
    -   Analgesics (NSAIDs) for pain.
    -   Cold compress for face.
    -   Review 1 week after the injury.

4. Reasons for mechanical preparation of root canals:

    -   Removal of vital pulp tissue from the canals
    -   Removal of necrotic tissues and microorganisms
    -   Removal of infected dentine
    -   Creating a space that can be adequately irrigated and filled

5. EDTA (ethylenediaminetetraacetic acid) is a chelator and a neutral or slightly alkaline solution. It is used inside the canal to help

remove the inorganic parts of the smear layer. EDTA has no antimicrobial effects but weakens the cell membrane, allowing other antimicrobial agents to attack the cell walls.

6. Four types of endodontic sealers:
    - Zinc oxide eugenol
    - Calcium hydroxide
    - Resin
    - Calcium silicate

7. Indications for apicectomy:
    - Presence of post inside the canal where it's removal can cause fracture of the root
    - Biopsy of the apical lesion

    Contraindications for apicectomy:
    - Inadequate orthograde endodontic present
    - Proximity of the nerve to the apex

8. The advantages of Crown-Down technique:
    - Allows irrigating solution to be used in the coronal part early on

- Prevents extrusion of infected tissue through the apex
- Helps to maintain the working length

9. Four ways to prevent instrument fracture:
   - Lubricate the canal using irrigation solution
   - Avoid excessive apical pressure when using the instruments
   - Discard deformed instruments
   - Use NiTi files with an auto reserve motor

10. As the irrigation solutions used in endodontics have poor surface tension and also air trapped at the canal can prevent complete irrigation, agitating the solution can be useful. This can be done manually using a side venting irrigation needle or Gutta percha point or it can be machine operated.

11. Four factors that can improve outcome of endodontic treatment:
    - The absence of periapical radiolucency before the start of the treatment
    - No voids present in the root fillings

- The root filling extending within 2 mm of the radiographic apex
- A satisfactory coronal restoration

12. Zip and elbow happens when an instrument is trying to straighten a curved canal. An hourglass shape is formed with the narrow part being the elbow and the flared apical part the zip. This makes it hard to shape the apical part of the root effectively.

13. Apical gauging refers to measuring the diameter of apical constriction. This is important as it helps decide the size of the Master Apical File. It also ensures that the taper of the final preparation extends all the way to the terminus of the canal.

14. Glide Path refers to straight line access to the apical region of the root canal. This would allow better access, and therefore more effective cleaning, shaping, irrigation and obturation of the root canal.

15. The four properties of ideal endodontic filling material:

- Nontoxic
- Radiopaque
- Adhesive
- Bactericidal

16. Two main aims of obturation:

- To prevent reinfection of the canal with bacteria/ exudate from coronal and apical ends
- To seal the remaining bacteria within the canal

17. Internal root resorption is an inflammatory process taking place inside the pulp and affecting the dentine and cementum. It forms a well-demarcated defect within the pulp with a symmetrical shape. Teeth affected by internal root resorption are vital or partially vital and the resorption may heal after endodontic therapy.

External root resorption starts on the surface of the root. It is often observed in teeth affected by trauma or moved during orthodontic treatment. External root resorptions are irregular in outline. Teeth affected by external root resorption can be vital or non-vital.

18. Three indications for use of systemic antibiotics in endodontic:
- Febrile patient
- Cellulitis
- Lymphadenopathy

19. Four techniques for removal of separated endodontic instruments:
- Masserann kit
- Hedstrom files
- Ultrasonic endodontic instruments
- Steiglitz forceps

20. Three properties of calcium hydroxide:
- Bacteriostatic and bactericidal
- Radiopaque
- Compatible with bonding materials

21. Reactionary dentine: a type of tertiary dentine which is secreted by post-mitotic odontoblast cells in response to mild stimulus (i.e. early caries/ mild abrasion)

Reparative dentine: a type of tertiary dentine secreted by new odontoblast cells in response to strong stimulus.

22. Periapical granuloma:

> This is a mass of granulation tissue, found at the apex of a tooth with pulpal infection. This is a well-circumscribed round radiolucency with a radiopaque border. This lesion is often less than 10mm in size.

Periapical cyst (Radicular cyst):

> This is an inflammatory odontogenic cyst, from the Rests of Mallases. It is often associated with the apex of non-vital maxillary central incisors. This is a well-defined round radiolucency with a radiopaque border, similar to periapical granuloma but larger than 10 mm in size.

23. Three anatomical landmarks mistaken for periapical lesions:
- Mental foramen
- Nasopalatine foramen
- Surgical scars (i.e. from apicectomy)

24. In ankylosis tooth becomes locked in cancellous bone. This is the result of Replacement Resorption which destroys the cementum and alveolar bone. This process of resorption causes the bone to be deposited directly within the resorbed tooth structure. The lack of periodontal ligament and the irregular nature of resorption leads to ankylosis and the lack of mobility of the tooth.

25. Four common causes for persistence of periapical disease:
- Inadequate cleaning of the canals
- Missed lateral canals
- Presence of calcified canals
- Inadequate apical or coronal seals

26. Three advantages of rubber dam:
- Preventing contamination of the canals by saliva
- Reducing risk of inhaling endodontic instruments
- Better visibility

27. Pulp polyp (Hyperplastic pulpitis) presents as a pinkish soft tissue mass, extruding from often long-standing dental cavities. The polyp consists of granulation tissue, connective tissue and blood supply and it is covered with epithelium. The treatment for pulp polyp includes Endodontic therapy or extraction of the tooth.

28. Two clinical situations where pulp testing could be indicated:

- In examination of traumatised teeth
- Before placing large restorations or preparing a tooth for fixed prosthetics

29. EPT (Electric Pulp Tester) is a battery-operated device which produces a pulsating electrical stimulus. The objective is to stimulate A-delta fibres in the pulp-dentine complex by applying the electrical current to the tooth surface. A positive response includes patient feeling a warm or tingling sensation from the tooth.

30. MTA (Mineral Trioxide Aggregate) is an endodontic cement, containing tricalcium silicate, tricalcium alluminate and bismuth oxide. MTA can be used in treatments such as apicectomy and repair of the perforation of the pulp chamber.

5 Dental Materials: Questions

1. Why is it important to shake the alginate powder before mixing it with water? And what is the ideal water temperature when mixing alginate?

2. Explain the terms "Syneresis" and "Imbition" with regard to alginate impressions.

3. What ingredient in alginate reacts with sodium to reduce the setting time of the impression?

4. Name two advantages and two disadvantages of alginate impression material.

5. Name two advantages of Polyether impression materials over alginate.

6. What are the effects of Polysaccharide and Calcium salt in alginate composition?

7. In what type of elastomer the reaction between monomers and alkyl silicate releases ethyl alcohol?

8. Name two advantages and two disadvantages of polyvinyl siloxane.

9. Explain the difference between "Mucodisplacive" and "Mucostatic" impression techniques.

10. Name two main types of base metal alloys and what is their advantage over gold?

11. Explain the terms "Elastic modulus" and "Stress" in relation to dental materials.

12. What type of dental cement works by forming ionic bond at tooth-cement interface?

13. Name two advantages and two disadvantages of using composite as a cement material.

14. What is the problem with having Gamma2 in amalgam and describe two ways to reduce the amount of Gamma2 in dental amalgam.

15. What are the roles of zinc and tin in dental amalgam?

16. Name three advantages and three disadvantages of dental amalgam.

17. Name four factors affecting light polymerisation of composite dental material.

18. Explain the different between "Auto-polymerisation" and "Light polymerisation" in composite dental material.

19. Name three advantages and three disadvantages of composite dental material.

20. Describe the three steps in Total Etch Technique in dentine bonding.

21. Glass Ionomer Cement contains Fluoroaluminosilicate glass and two other main ingredients. Name these two.

22. Name two advantages and two disadvantages of Glass Ionomer Cements.

23. Describe three patient selection criteria for placing fissure sealants.

24. What factors affect the onset and duration of injectable local anaesthetics?

25. Name three self/light cure resin materials that can be used in construction of temporary crown/ Bridge.

6 Dental Materials: Answers

1. Shaking the alginate powder before mixing helps to incorporate the surface layer which has absorbed moisture from the environment. The ideal water temperature is 23°C.

2. Syneresis: This refers to extraction of liquid from a gel and can cause shrinkage of alginate impressions.

   Imbition: This refers to taking up moisture from the environment which causes expansion of alginate impressions.

3. Calcium salt

4. Advantages of alginate:

   - Hydrophillic
   - Short setting time

Disadvantages of alginate:
- Should be poured quickly
- Can only be poured once

5. The two advantages of Polyether impression materials over alginate are:
   - Polyethers have better tear resistance than alginate
   - Polyethers have better dimensional stability than alginates

6. Polysaccharide is responsible for irreversible setting of the alginate. Calcium salt reacts with sodium to slow down the setting time

7. Condensation silicone

8. Advantages of polyvinyl siloxane:

   - Dimensionally stable
   - Can be poured multiple times

   Disadvantages of polyvinyl siloxane:
   - Hydrophobic
   - Low tear resistance

9. Mucodisplacive impression technique is taking impression of the mucosa under load (during function). The aim of the impression is to gain maximum support from flabby ridge. Impression compound, high viscosity alginate and elastomers can be used for mucodisplacive impressions.

   Mucostatic impression technique is taking impression of undisplaced mucosa (Mucosa at resting position). The aim of the impression is to maximise retention by getting support from the other areas of the arch. Zinc oxide and eugenol and low viscosity alginate can be used for Mucostatic impressions.

10. Cobalt chromium and nickel chromium. The elastic modulus of these alloys are twice that of the gold.

11. Elastic modulus is the measure of the rigidity of the material. It is the ratio of tensile stress to tensile strain.

    Stress refers to the internal force set up in reaction to and opposite the applied force. Stress can be classified as tensile, compressive or shear.

12. Glass Ionomer Cement works by chelation of carboxyl group in acid with calcium or phosphate in enamel and dentine.

13. Advantages of composite as cement:

- Good compressive and tensile strength
- Insoluble in oral environment

Disadvantages of composite as cement:

- Polymerisation shrinkage
- Sensitivity to moisture

14. Gamma2 containing amalgam has low tensile strength and is more prone to dimensional changes and microleakage.

Gamme2 phase can be reduced by reducing the amount of silver and adding more copper. This can be done in two ways:

- Using a mixture of lathe-cut and spherical amalgam (Admix)
- Producing an alloy with high copper content (12-35%)

15. Zinc increases wettability (the ability of the material to flow over a surface) and tin slows down the setting time.

16. Advantages:

- Easy to use
- Strong
- High wear resistance

Disadvantages:

- Initial microleakage
- Doesn't provide insulation for the tooth
- Poor aesthetic

17. The four factors are:
- Filler loading
- Particle sizes
- The distance between light source and restoration

18. In auto-polymerisation an addition polymerisation occurs due to the mixing of benzoic peroxide and a tertiary amine which releases free radicals.

In light polymerisation, diketone when exposed to light (460-470 wavelength) reacts with a tertiary amine, leading to free radical initiation and setting of the material.

19. Advantages of composite:

- Can bond to the tooth and strengthen it
- No need to create undercuts for restoration
- Low thermal conductivity (provides insulation for the tooth)

Disadvantages of composite:

- Polymerisation shrinkage
- Technique sensitive
- Thermal expansion up to three times higher than the tooth

20. The three steps in Total Etch Technique are:

Step I: Acid etch, phosphoric acid (conditioner) applied to the cut dentine for 15 seconds. This removes the smear layer, demineralises the top 2-5 microns of dentine and opens 20-30 nanometre channels around the collagen fibrils. The acid and the dissolved smear layer are removed using air spray.

Step II: Primer (Wetting agent with HEMA) is applied to the area. This is a bifunctional material both hydrophilic to bond to the dentine and hydrophobic to bond to the adhesive.

Step III: Adhesive resin is applied to stabilise the hybrid layer and form resin tags in exposed dentine tubules. The tags will seal the dentine surface even if mechanical bonding fails.

21. Polyacrylic acid and tartaric acid

22. Advantages of Glass Ionomer Cement:
  • Durable adhesion to tooth surface under moist conditions
  • Releases fluoride

Disadvantages of Glass Ionomer Cement:
  • Low compressive and flexural strength.

- Releases water during setting which affects its dimensional stability.

23. Three patient selection criteria for Fissure sealants are:
- Previous experience of caries
- Good patient cooperation and moisture control
- Medically compromised patients

24. Local anaesthetic solutions with more acidic pH have slower onset. The duration of the anaesthesia depends on the ability of the anaesthetic molecule to bind to the protein in the nerve's sodium channels.

25. Polymethyl methacrylate, Polyethyl methacrylate, Bis acryl composite

7 Restorative and Prosthodontics: Questions

1. Describe the difference between "Centric Occlusion" and "Centric Relation".

2. Explain the term "Balanced Occlusion".

3. What is "Terminal Hinge Axis"?

4. Name four possible complications of endodontic treatment of crowned teeth.

5. Describe the "Ferrule Effect".

6. Describe four advantages of using temporary crowns.

7. Name two indications and two contraindications for porcelain crowns.

8. Explain the difference between "Functional Cusp" and "Non-functional Cusp".

9. Describe the Kennedy classification for removable partial dentures.

10. Name six muscles that can affect peripheral flanges of a complete denture.

11. What is "Post Dam"?

12. What material is most suitable for a clasp in an undercut of 0.75 mm?

13. What is the function of a "Facebow"?

14. Name three major connectors in removable lower partial dentures.

15. Describe two functions of rests in removable partial dentures.

16. Explain the differences between a "3-arm clasp" and a "Ring clasp" in removable partial dentures.

17. Explain two indications for using Ring clasps in removable partial dentures.

18. What problems with complete dentures make it difficult for patients to pronounce the letters D, S and T?

19. Describe three types of porosity that can occur in acrylic resins of dentures.

20. Describe three types of tooth wear.

21. Explain four steps in monitoring and management of tooth wear.

22. Describe the terms "Resistance" and "Retention" in relation to conservative dentistry.

23. Explain the functions of "Retraction Cords".

24. Describe four indications for "Copy Dentures".

25. Name three advantages and three disadvantages of "Immediate Dentures".

26. Describe four characteristics of "Every" Dentures.

27. Explain the function of RPI (Rest, Plate, I-Bar clasp) in mandibular distal extension saddle.

28. Describe four steps in designing an Anterior Resin Retained Bridge.

29. Name four intrinsic factors causing tooth discolouration.

30. Describe the "Ellis Classification" of complete fractures of the teeth.

8 Restorative and Prosthodontics: Answers

1. Centric Occlusion is the position of maximum intercuspation. It is the habitual bite and a static position.

   Centric Relation is the position of mandible to maxilla when condyle is at terminal hinge axis/ position of mandible to maxilla when condylar head is at the most superior part of glenoid fossa. This is a reproducible and dynamic position.

2. This refers to balancing contact in all excursion of mandible to provide complete dentures with increased stability. This occlusion does not apply to natural dentition.

3. Terminal Hinge Axis is an imaginary line around which mandible rotates within the saggital plane.

4. The four complications of endodontic treatment of crowned teeth are:

    - Difficulty with accessing the canals
    - Fracture of the porcelain crowns
    - Weakening the cement
    - Rubber dam clasps causing damage to the crown

5. Ferrule Effect refers to a 2 mm band of supra-gingival tooth structure which helps reduce the risk of tooth fracture after crowning a root filled tooth/ A band of cast metal around the coronal surface of the tooth.

6. The advantages of temporary crowns are:

    - Help protect the pulp
    - Restore the function of the tooth
    - Help maintain the position of the tooth
    - Prevent over-eruption of the opposing tooth

7. Indications for porcelain crowns:
- Large inadequate anterior restorations
- Severely discoloured anterior teeth

Contraindications for porcelain crowns:
- Insufficient tooth tissue available
- Edge to edge occlusion

8. Functional Cusp (Supporting cusp/ working cusp) refers to buccal cusps of mandibular posterior teeth and palatal cusps of maxillary posterior teeth.

Non-functional Cusp (non-working cusp/non-centric cusp) refers to buccal cusps of maxillary posterior teeth and lingual cusps of mandibular posterior teeth.

9. Kennedy classification:

Kennedy class I: Bilateral free end saddle

Kennedy class II: Unilateral free end saddle

Kennedy class III: Posterior bounded saddle

Kennedy class IV: Anterior bounded saddle

10. The six muscles are:
- Geniohyoid
- Mylohyiod
- Orbicularis oris
- Mentalis
- Palatoglossus
- Palatopharyngeus

11. Post Dam refers to raised lip on the posterior border of upper complete dentures which supresses the soft tissue to produce a border seals.

12. A gold clasp is most suitable as the high modulus of elasticity of gold means that it can engage a deep undercut without permanent deformation.

13. Facebow allows placing the maxillary cast on a semi-adjustable articulator at a fixed anatomical landmark.

14. The three major connectors are:
- Lingual bar
- Sublingual bar
- Lingual plate

15. Rests direct the forces along the long axis of the tooth. They also provide indirect retention in bilateral free end saddles and anterior bounded saddles.

16. A 3-arm clasp is a single arm clasp with occlusal rest and a reciprocal arm. A ring clasp is a round clasp and reciprocation is achieved from the rigid arm being on the opposite side of the tooth from the retentive tip.

17. Ring clasps are suitable when there is a large undercut near the saddle and around tilted molars.

18. Alterations of palatal contour, incorrect overjet, incorrect overbite

19. The three types of porosity are:

- Contraction porosity: Caused by insufficient acrylic or insufficient pressure during curing. This leads to voids throughout the denture base.
- Gaseous porosity: Caused if the temperature of the dough is raised above the boiling point of the monomer. This leads to well-defined

defects on the thicker parts of the denture, especially the lingual flanges of lower dentures.

- Granular porosity: Caused by the loss of monomer during preparation. This leads to white and opaque surfaces on the thinner parts of the denture.

20. The three types of tooth wear are:

Erosion: This refers to tooth wear caused by acid. Erosion could be due to intrinsic acids (i.e. gastric acid) or extrinsic acid (such as carbonated drinks and citrus fruit)

Attrition: This is tooth wear caused by tooth-to-tooth or tooth-to-restoration contact. Attrition is most common in patients with bruxism or those who clench their teeth.

Abrasion: This is tooth wear caused by extrinsic sources such as tooth brushing

21. The four steps in monitoring and management of tooth wear are:

- Using clinical photographs and study models to monitor tooth wear
- Application of fluoride varnish to the affected area
- Restoration of the affected area with adhesive materials
- Use of night guards to prevent further tooth wear

22. Resistance in restorations refer to type of cavity design which allows tooth and its restoration to tolerate functional forces.

Retention in restorations refers to the design of the cavity walls to prevent the restoration getting dislodged from the cavity under functional forces.

23. Retraction Cords help to push gingival tissue away from the preparation margins of extra coronal restorations and they also help with haemostasis of gingival tissues if necessary. Retraction cords can be braided or woven cottons. Some are impregnated with astringents such as aluminium sulphate or ferric sulphate and others are non-impregnated.

24. The four indications for Copy Dentures are:
- Occlusal wear or loss of retention in an otherwise satisfactory denture
- Replacement of immediate dentures
- To make a spare denture
- Loss of denture base material

25. Advantages of Immediate Dentures:
- Provides aesthetic and functional support by replacing the natural tooth/teeth immediately
- Helps patient get used to wearing a denture
- Helps maintain the tooth position

Disadvantages of Immediate Dentures:
- Quick loss of retention due to alveolar bone resorption post extraction
- A reline, rebase or a new denture may be required within few months post extraction

- Lack of trial stage means patient can't see what the denture would look like

26. The characteristics of "Every" Dentures are:
    - Designed to replace teeth in multiple bounded edentulous areas in maxilla
    - All connector borders are 3 mm away from the gingival margins
    - There are point contacts between false teeth and abutment teeth to reduce lateral stress
    - Posterior wing stops are added to prevent distal drifting of posterior teeth

27. In the RPI system, the tip of the I-Bar clasp contacts the most prominent part of the buccal surface of the abutment tooth. This means that when under occlusal force, the saddle sinks, the tip of the clasp moves away from the tooth, reducing the stress on the tooth.

28. The four steps in designing an Anterior Resin Retained Bridge are:

- Ovate pontic for better aesthetics
- Maximum retainer coverage for better retention
- Retainer of 0.7 mm thickness
- Minimal intercuspal position contact

29. The intrinsic factors causing tooth discolouration are:

- Fluorosis
- Root resorption
- Amelogenesis imperfect
- Tetracycline staining

30. The Ellis Classifications of tooth fracture are:

Ellis I: Fracture involving enamel only and often symptomless

Ellis II: Fracture involving enamel and dentine. This can cause sensitivity and pain to touch

Ellis III: Fracture involving enamel, dentine and pulp causing significant pain and sensitivity.

9 Oral Surgery: Questions

1. Name three local haemostatic agents.

2. Name five risk factors for Dry Socket (Alveolar osteitis) and how is this condition treated?

3. What are three possible causes of a non-healing socket after extraction?

4. What causes pericoronitis? What are some of its signs and symptoms?

5. Name five indications for extraction of a third molar according to the NICE (National Institute for Health and Care Excellence) guidelines.

6. What are the risks of temporary and permanent damage to Inferior dental nerve and lingual nerve during extractions of lower third molars?

7. Describe four radiographic signs of Inferior dental nerve being close to the apex of a lower third molar.

8. Describe three factors that are considered during assessment of impacted third molars.

9. Name five possible complications of third molar extraction.

10. How would you manage a root fracture during extraction?

11. Describe the "Winter's Line" Index.

12. Name four possible signs of a mandibular fracture.

13. Describe three circumstances in which Open reduction and internal fixation (ORIF) is indicated in treatment of a fractured mandible.

14. Describe four characteristics of a zygomatic fracture.

15. Explain the differences between Le fort I, II and III fractures.

16. What is the most common cause of a fractured orbital floor?

17. What fracture is also known as "Bucket handle fracture"?

18. Name four risk factors for Oro-antral Communication (OAC).

19. Name four signs and symptoms of Oro-antral Fistula (OAF).

20. Name two types of flaps that can be used in treatment of OAF.

21. What is the most common cause of Maxillary tuberosity fracture?

22. What causes "Surgical Emphysema" and how is it resolved?

23. Name three materials used in production of absorbable sutures.

24. Describe the differences between Incisional biopsies and Excisional biopsies.

25. Name three types of elevators used in dental extractions.

10 Oral Surgery: Answers

1. The three local haemostatic agents:
    - Oxidised cellulose (Surgicell)
    - Collagen sponge (Heamocollagen)
    - Gelatine sponge (Spongostan)

2. Risk factors for Dry Socket include:
    - Smoking after extraction
    - Traumatic extraction
    - Oral contraceptive pill
    - Excessive local anaesthetic containing vasoconstrictor
    - Extractions of mandibular third molars

    Management of Dry Socket:
    - Reassure the patient
    - Irrigate the socket with saline/ Chlorhexidine
    - Place Alvogyl inside the socket

- Advise the patient to rinse with salty mouthwash/ take analgesics when necessary
- Review the patient in 5-7 days

3. The causes for non-healing sockets:
   - Osteomyelitis
   - Oral cancer
   - Retained root

4. Operculum extending over a partially erupted third molar can get infected by bacteria (Fusobacterium/ Bacteroids) or traumatised by the opposing tooth. Some of the signs and symptoms include: Pain, bad taste, trismus and in severe cases pyrexia.

5. The indications for extraction of third molars according to NICE guidelines:
   - Two episodes of severe pericoronitis where patient would need antibiotics and one very severe episode of periocoronitis
   - Untreatable caries
   - Untreatable pulpal/ periapical disease
   - Cellulitis

- Abscess

6. For Inferior dental nerve:
    - Risk of temporary damage: 5-10%
    - Risk of permanent damage: 0.3- 0.6%

   For lingual nerve:

    - Risk of temporary damage: 11%
    - Risk of permanent damage: 0.6%

7. Radiographic signs that the inferior dental nerve is close to the apex of lower third molar:
    - Loss of tramline
    - Narrowing of tramline
    - Sudden change in the direction of tramline
    - Radiolucent band across the tramline

8. Three factors considered in assessment of impacted third molars:
    - Angulation of the third molar
    - The relationship of the third molar with the adjacent second molar
    - Depth of impaction and the overlying tissue

9. The complications of third molar extraction:
- Pain
- Swelling
- Infection
- Fracture of the tooth/ retained root
- Damage to the nerve

10. To manage a root fracture:
- Inform the patient that part of the root is broken.
- Take a periapical radiograph to assess:
  - The retained root can be left if:
    - Patient refuses further surgery.
    - Less than 1/3 of the root is left.
    - There are no signs of infection associated with the retained root.
    - Retained root has not been displaced.
- Retained root can be removed by surgical extraction.

11. "Winter's Line" Index: An index for assessing the position and depth of lower third molars. Three lines (White, red and amber) are drawn on a periapical radiograph or oral panoramic tomograph (OPT).

- The white line is drawn at the occlusal level of the lower first and second molar, extending over to the third molar.
- The amber line is drawn at the alveolar crest of the lower first and second molar, extending distally to follow the Internal oblique ridge.
- The red line is perpendicular from the amber line to the possible point of application mesial on the third molar. It indicates the amount of bone that needs to be removed for extraction of third molar. If the red line is 5 mm or more, extraction under general anaesthesia is indicated.

12. Four signs of mandibular fracture:

- Pain and swelling
- Paraesthesia
- Step deformity
- Pain on deviation

13. Three circumstances in which ORIF is indicated in treatment of fractures:
- In severe injuries causing displacement
- In edentulous or semi-edentulous jaw
- In multiple fractures of midface

14. Four characteristics of zygomatic fracture:
- Flattening of check bones
- Diplopia
- Paraesthesia of infra-orbital nerve
- Limited lateral excursion

15. The differences between Le fort fractures:

Le fort I: Teeth bearing part of maxilla is detached.

Le fort II: Pyramidal fracture of maxilla, involving nasal bone and infra-orbital rims.

Le fort III: Affects nasal bone and zygomatic-frontal suture. The whole of the maxilla is detached from the base of the skull.

16. Interpersonal trauma on the left-hand side.

17. Bilateral parasymphyseal fracture.

18. Four risk factors for OAC:
- Extraction of maxillary molars
- Maxillary tumours
- Osteomyelitis
- Extraction of a lone standing maxillary molar

19. Four signs and symptoms of OAF:
- The fistula is larger than 5 mm.
- Food and drink enter the nose.
- Patient has difficulty smoking.
- Patient complains of bad breath.

20. The two types of flaps are:

The Buccal advancement flap:

> The OAC is removed and a broad-based trapezoid mecoperiosteal flap is created. The flap is advanced and sutured to the palatine tissue. These types of flaps are more suitable for smaller communications (less than 5 mm). The flap is less likely to get traumatised during the healing process, but the

procedure can lead to a shallow buccal sulcus, interfering with future prosthodontics treatments.

The Palatal-rotation advancement flap:

A full thickness mucoperiosteal flap is raised, leaving about 5 mm of palatal marginal gingiva to avoid periodontal damage. The flap is rotated, advanced and sutured to the buccal tissue. These flaps are more suitable for larger communications (more than 5 mm) due to better blood supply. They however are more difficult to perform.

21. Extraction of maxillary molars.

22. Surgical Emphysema is collection of air below the subcutaneous tissue. The air can go under the flap if a high-speed hand piece is used for example during surgical extractions. This is often a benign condition which resolves in 3-10 days. Some clinicians may prescribe a course of antibiotics to prevent infection of the subcutaneous tissue by oral bacteria.

23. Materials used in production of absorbable sutures:
- Polyglycolic acid
- Polyglactin
- Catgut (Sheep intestine!)

24. Differences between Excisional and Incisional biopsies:

Incisional biopsy is used to remove a representative sample of the lesion and part of its surrounding healthy tissue for diagnosis and treatment. This biopsy is the method of choice in suspected malignancies.

Excisional biopsy aims to remove the lesion completely for definitive diagnosis and treatment. This biopsy is the method of choice when the lesion is very likely to be non-malignant.

25. Three types of elevators:
- Couplands
- Cryers (left and right)
- Warwick James (left and right)

11 Oral Medicine:
Questions

1. What is the most common cause of Trigeminal neurolgia?

2. Describe four signs and symptoms of Migranous neurolgia (Cluster Headache) and how is this condition treated?

3. Name two Tempromandibular Joint (TMJ) ligaments.

4. Name five factors that could lead to Burning Mouth Syndrome (Oral dysaesthesia) and describe three symptoms of this condition.

5. Name four buccal spaces in the head.

6. Describe five signs of spreading infection.

7. How would you diagnose Herpetiform ulcers? Name four risk factors for Aphthous ulcerations.

8. Name three risk factors for Angular cheilitis.

9. Name three pre-disposing factors for Herpes labialis (Cold sore) and how is this condition treated?

10. What cells are identified in the smear test from vesicles in diagnosis of Primary herpetic gingivostomatitis?

11. Describe the difference between primary and secondary Sjögren's syndrome.

12. Name four investigations used in diagnosis of Sjögren's syndrome.

13. Name two saliva substitutes that can be prescribed to patients with dry mouth.

14. Name five differential diagnoses for white patches in the mouth.

15. Name four differential diagnoses for lumps on the palate.

16. Describe two viral infections that can affect salivary glands.

17. What is Sialolithiasis?

18. Name two benign tumours of salivary glands.

19. "Saw tooth rete process" and "Civatte bodies" are histological findings associated with which autoimmune disease?

20. Describe four histological signs of Dysplasia.

21. What is a "Ranula"?

22. Name two acute and two chronic types of candidiasis.

23. Explain the differences between fibrous and vascular epulides.

24. What is the most common odontogenic cyst? Describe four of its characteristics.

25. Describe five characteristics of Dentigerous cysts.

26. Name two conditions responsible for depapillation of the dorsal surface of the tongue.

27. Explain the main histological difference between Pemphigus and Pemphigoid.

28. What causes Submucus Fibrosis? Describe four of its characteristics.

29. What disease are caused by HHV3, HHV4 and HHV8?

30. Name five pre-cancerous lesions.

12 Oral medicine: Answers

1. The most common cause of Trigeminal neurolgia is the compression of trigeminal nerve in the region of Dorsal root entry zone (DREZ) by a blood vessel.

2. Four signs of Migranous neurolgia:
   - This condition affects one side of the face.
   - Causes flushing of the neck
   - Causes eye to water on the affected side.
   - Causes nasal congestion on the affected side.

   The treatment of choice is sumatriptan.

3. Two TMJ ligaments:

- Sphenomandibular ligament
- Stylomandibular ligament

4. Factors leading to Burning Mouth Syndrome:
   - Parafunction
   - Allergic reaction to monomers used in acrylic dentures
   - Depression
   - ACE inhibitors

   Symptoms of Burning Mouth Syndrome:
   - Dry mouth
   - Numbness of the tip of the tongue
   - Bitter/metallic taste in the mouth

5. The four buccal spaces:
   - Submasseteric space
   - Pterygomandibular space
   - Infratemporal space
   - Parotid space

6. Five signs of spreading infection:
   - Increased pain
   - Rapid swelling
   - Fever
   - Increased pulse rate

- Uncontrolled diabetes

7. Herpetiform ulcers are pin-head size ulcers (1-2 mm), presenting in crops of 100 or more on non-keratinised tissue. They heal within 1-2 weeks.

    Risk factors for aphthous ulceration:
    - Stress
    - Smoking cessation
    - Family history
    - Vitamin B12 deficiency

8. Three risk factors for angular cheilitis:
    - Iron deficiency anaemia
    - Reduced Occlusal vertical dimension (OVD)
    - Diabetes

9. Pre-disposing factors for herpes labialis:
    - Stress
    - Sunlight
    - Low immunity

The treatment includes application of acyclovir cream 5% to the lesion, five times a day for 5 days.

10. Tzanck cells

11. Primary Sjögren's syndrome includes xerostomia and xerophthalmia.

Secondary Sjögren's syndrome is accompanied by autoimmune connective tissue disorder such as Rheumatoid arthritis or systemic lupus erythematous in addition to xerostomia and xerophthalmia.

12. Four investigations in diagnosis of Sjögren's syndrome:
- Sialometry
- Labial gland biopsy
- Sialography
- Schirmer test

13. Two saliva substitutes:
- Carboxymethyl cellulose-based, e.g., Luborant
- Mucin-based, e.g., Saliva Orthana

14. Five differential diagnoses for white patches in the mouth:
- Candida
- Papilloma
- Leukoplakia
- Whaite sponge neavi
- Burns

15. Four differential diagnoses for lumps on the palate:
- Tori
- Impacted tooth
- Denture granuloma
- Squamous cell carcinoma

16. Two viral infections affecting salivary glands:

Mumps:

> This is an infection by paramyoxyvirus. It can spread by direct contacts or through droplets. Mumps causes fever, malaise and painful unilateral or bilateral swelling of the parotid glands. In adults mumps can affect the central nervous system and the gonads.

Secondary to HIV:

This infection causes bilateral enlargement of parotid glands. The symptoms are similar to those of Sjögren's syndrome and it is diagnosed through GIV serology.

17. Sialolithiasis is the most common salivary gland disease, affecting the submandibular gland in 80% of the cases. This condition is caused by the formation and retention of salivary calculus (hard and yellow with a ring structure made of calcium and phosphate) inside the ducts in the glands. Sialolithiasis causes painful swelling of the salivary gland at meal times (in response to smell and taste of food). The diagnosis is aided by plain radiographs and ultrasound imaging.

18. Two benign tumours of salivary glands:
- Wharton's tumour
- Pleomorphic adenoma

19. Lichen planus

20. Four histological signs of Dysplasia:

- Nuclear pleomorphism
- Premature keratinisation
- Supra-basal mitosis
- Tear-drop shaped rete process

21. A Ranula is an extravasation mucocele which can be found on lower labial mucosa, buccal mucosa or floor of the mouth. It is caused by breakage of salivary ducts through trauma which then leads to saliva leaking into the surrounding connective tissue. A granulation tissue capsule is then formed which is filled with mucin and macrophages. If Ranula pierces the mylohyoid muscle and goes into the submandibular space, it would be known as a "Plunging Ranula".

Ranulas are more common in infants and younger people and often spontaneously resolved.

22. Acute candidiasis:
- Thrush (Pseudomembranous)
- Atrophic (Erythromatous)

Chronic candidiasis:

- Angular chelitis
- Median Rhomboid glossitis

23. Fibrous epulides are similar to gingival polyps. They have a core of dense collagenous tissue and are covered by epithelium. They can get traumatised and ulcerated easily. This type of epulides often caused by trauma or faulty restorations.

Vascular epulides (e.g. Pregnancy granuloma) have a core of vascular tissue. These are red and fleshy gingival swellings that bleed easily. These epulides are often caused by hormonal changes during pregnancy or puberty.

24. Amleblastoma:

- An slow-growing lesion, affecting the posterior mandible
- More common in patients of African origin
- Causes bone expansion, teeth displacement, root resorption and pain
- It can be categorised as Follicular or Plexiform

25. Five characteristics of Dentigerous cysts:
- Benign developmental odontogenic cysts
- Derives from Reduced Enamel Epithelium (REE)
- 3-4 mm in size, enclosing the crown of the tooth
- Lined with stratifies squamous epithelium
- Most commonly affects mandibular third molars

26. Anaemia and Xerostomia

27. In Pemphigus, intra-epithelial lesions are caused by binding of the IgG to the glycogen on hemi desmosomes. This binding weakens the intra-cellular connection in epithelial layer, causing intra-epithelial blisters.

In Pemphigoid, sub-epithelial lesions are caused by the binding of auto-antibodies to antigens in basal cell membrane. This activates leucocytes and complements, causing damage to the basement membrane and formation of sub-epithelial blisters.

28. This condition is caused by Betal nut, Paan or chewing tobacco.

- Orange/brown teeth
- Pale mucosa
- Limited mouth opening
- Mucosa feels firm on palpation

29. The diseases are:

- HHV3 (Zoster) is responsible for chickenpox and shingles.
- HHV4 (Epstein barr) can cause Glandular fever, Burkitt's lymphoma and Hairy leukoplakia.
- HHV8 can cause Kaposi's sarcoma.

30. Five pre-cancerous lesions:

- Erythroplakia
- Hyperplastic candida
- Erosive lichen planus
- Actinic chelitis
- Submucus Fibrosis

13 Peadodontics & Orthodontics: Questions

1. Name four causes for missing central incisors in children.

2. Describe five differences between deciduous and permanent teeth.

3. What is "Subluxation" and how is it treated?

4. What is the indication for Indirect Pulp Capping in paediatric patients and what material is commonly used for this procedure?

5. Describe the "Angle's Classification" of malocclusion.

6. Explain four components of IOTN (Index of Treatment Need) grade 4.

7. Name two functional appliances used in orthodontics and two of the dental changes they can make.

8. Explain the terms "Balance Enforced" and "Compensate Enforced" extractions.

9. What is the prevalence of impacted maxillary canines? Describe the Parallax Technique in assessing the position of an impacted canine.

10. Describe four causes of an Anterior Open Bite (AOB).

11. What is a "Crossbite" and name three components of an Upper Removable Appliance (URA) that can be used in correction of an anterior crossbite.

12. Describe five indications for early orthodontic referral.

13. What is the "Leeway Space"?

14. What are the benefits of Fluoride Varnish 22,600 ppm application? When is it contra-indicated?

15. Which fluoride mouthwashes can be prescribed for patients of 8 years of age or older?

16. Describe two effects of fluoride on teeth pre-eruption and two of its effects post-eruption.

17. What is the prevalence of Hypodontia in primary and permanent dentition? What are the two most commonly missing permanent teeth?

18. Explain the term "Invaginated tooth" or "dens invaginatus".

19. Name three factors that can be responsible for chronological enamel defects.

20. Describe three radiographic findings associated with Dentinogenesis Imperfecta.

21. Describe four signs and symptoms associated with Primary Herpetic Gingivostomatitis. How is this condition managed?

22. Describe four indications and four contraindications for Fissure sealants.

23. Name two advantages and two disadvantages of using Stainless Steel Crowns (SSC) in treatment of paediatric patients.

24. Describe the difference between hypoplasia and hypocalcification in enamel defect.

25. Define the "Primate Space".

26. When are the root calcifications completed in primary and secondary dentitions?

27. Explain the terms "Modelling" and "Behaviour Shaping" in child behaviour management.

28. Describe four benefits of nitrous oxide inhalation sedation in treatment of child patients.

29. What is the first choice of anaesthetic solution for child patient and how much is often sufficient for anaesthetising primary teeth?

30. Describe four features associated with Non-Accidental Injuries (NAI) in children that could be detected by dental staff.

14 Peadodontics & Orthodontics: Answers

1. Four causes of missing central incisors:
   - Extracted/ Avulsed tooth
   - Supernumerary
   - Crowding
   - Congenitally missing teeth

2. Differences between deciduous and permanent teeth:
   - Deciduous teeth are smaller than permanent teeth.
   - The roots of deciduous teeth are shorter, weaker and lighter in colour than permanent teeth.
   - Enamel is thinner in deciduous teeth.
   - The enamel in deciduous teeth are more permeable than in permanent teeth.

- The pulp chambers in deciduous teeth are larger and with more prominent pulp horns.

3. Subluxation refers to the injury to the tooth-supporting tissue with increased mobility but no displacement. It is often accompanied by gingival bleeding.

Flexible splint can be used for two weeks if tooth is painful during function. Radiographic checks at four weeks, eight weeks and one year post injury helps to detect signs of infection or resorption.

4. Indirect Pulp Capping is indicated in deep carious lesions which are close to the pulp but without pulpal exposure. Hard-setting calcium hydroxide is used to encourage tertiary dentine formation at the base of the cavity.

5. Angle's Classifications of malocclusion:

Class I: The mesio-buccal cusp of maxillary first molar occludes with the buccal groove of the mandibular first molar. The facial profile is mesognathic.

Class II: The mesio-buccal cusp of maxillary first molar occludes mesial to the buccal grove of the mandibular first molar. The facial profile is retrognathic.

Division I:

First molars are in class II and central incisors are protruded.

Division II:

First molars are in class II and central incisors are retruded

Class III: The mesio-buccal cusp of maxillary first molars occludes distal to the buccal groove on mandibular first molar. The facial profile is prognathic.

6. Four components of IOTN grade 4:
   - Increased overjet greater than 6 mm but less than or equal to 9 mm.
   - Reversed overjet greater than 6 mm with no masticatory or speech problems.

- Severe contact point displacement greater than 4 mm
- Lateral or anterior open bite greater than 4 mm

7. Frankel and Twin block are two functional appliances and they can cause:
   - Palatal tipping of upper incisors
   - Preventing forward movement of maxillary molars

8. Balancing extraction refers to extraction of the same tooth on the opposite side of the same arch. This is to prevent centreline shift.

   Compensating extraction refers to extraction of an opposing tooth to prevent its over eruption.

9. Ectopic maxillary canines affect 2% of the population. In 85% of the cases canines are impacted palatally and in 15% buccally.

   In Parallax method, two periapical radiographs are taken at different angles to assess the position of the impacted canine. The first periapical radiograph is taken at a mesial horizontal angle which could show the crown of the canine overlapping the distal part of the central incisor. The second periapical radiograph is then taken at a more distal angle. In this radiograph the canine has either shift distally or mesially. If the canine shifts in the same direction as the tube, the tooth is placed palatally, but if it shifts in the opposite direction to the tube, it is placed buccally. SLOB: Same Lingual (palatal), Opposite Buccal.

10. Four causes of AOB:
    - Digit sucking
    - Increased lower face height
    - Localised failure of alveolar growth
    - Tongue thrust

11. A Crossbite refers to the discrepancy in the bucco-lingual relationship of the upper and lower teeth.

    A URA consists of Buccal Capping (to open the occlusion), Z springs (to push incisors forward) and Adam's Cribs on first molars (to help with retention).

12. Five indications for early orthodontic referral:
- Supplemental incisors
- Congenitally missing teeth
- Maxillary incisors in crossbite
- Impacted mandibular first molars
- Severe skeletal discrepancies

13. Leeway Space refers to the difference in size between the deciduous posterior teeth (C, D and E) and permanent canines and first and second premolars. After exfoliation of primary teeth, there is often a 2.5 mm space left in the maxilla and 1.5 mm space left in the mandible.

14. Biannual application of Fluoride Varnish 22,600 ppm can reduce the risk of caries in primary teeth by 33% and in permanent teeth by 46%.

The varnish is contra-indicated in Ulcerative gingivitis, stomatitis and in patients suffering from severe asthma.

15. The fluoride mouthwashes for patients of 8 years of age or older are:

- 0.2% Sodium fluoride mouthwash, used once a week
- 0.05% sodium fluoride mouthwash, used once a day

16. Pre eruption effects of fluoride:
    - Teeth with rounded cusps and shallow fissures
    - Larger enamel crystals which are less acid soluble

    Post eruption effects of fluoride:
    - Prevents glycolysis
    - Reduces demineralisation and encourages remineralisation

17. The prevalence of Hypodontia:
    - 0.1-0.9% in primary dentition
    - 3.5-6.5% in permanent dentition

    Third molars are the most commonly missing teeth followed by mandibular second premolars.

18. Invaginated tooth is an abnormality of the crown of the tooth caused by an invagination of enamel epithelium into the dental papilla during development. It sometimes presents as a deep cingulum pit on the palatal surface of maxillary lateral incisors.

19. Three factors responsible for chronological enamel defects:

- Chronic childhood diseases such as hypothyroidism, chronic renal disease and coeliac disease
- Use of tetracycline during pregnancy
- Excessive fluoride

20. Three radiographic findings associated with Dentinogenesis Imperfecta:
- Bulbous crowns
- Short and thin roots
- Pulp chambers obliterated with dentin depositions

21. Primary Herpetic Gingivostomatitis is caused by Herpesvirus hominis (HVH type I) and is transmitted through droplets. It affects children between two and five years of age. Fluid-filled vesicles appear on the gingiva, lips, tongue and buccal mucosa. The vesicle burst resulting in painful yellow ulcers. The condition also causes fever, malaise and cervical lymphadenopathy. The episode runs for 14 days and ulcers heal without scarring.

Management includes bed rest, keeping hydrated, paracetamol suspension for fever and using chlorhexidine mouthwash to prevent the secondary infection of the ulcers.

22. Indications for Fissure sealants:

- Previous caries experience in primary or permanent dentition
- Cooperative patient
- Medically compromised patient
- Deep or demineralised pits and fissures

Contraindications for Fissure sealants:

- Carious fissures
- Radiolucency visible on the bitewing radiographs indicating dentine caries
- Shallow pits and fissures
- Uncooperative patient/ inadequate isolation

23. Advantages of SSC:

- Durable
- Simple and quick procedure

Disadvantages of SSC:

- Poor aesthetics
- Not conservative

24. Enamel hypoplasia is caused by disturbance in ameloblastic function during amelogenesis. This is the failure of development of enamel matrix. Hypoplasia can lead to the lack of normal features in the tooth such as mamelons and cusps. The enamel can also be discoloured, thin and more prone to caries.

Enamel hypocalcification is caused by failure in the maturation of ameloblasts. The hypocalcified enamel has a chalky, white appearance and is porous, weak and less resistant to abrasion.

25. Primate Space is a naturally occurring space in primary dentition, mesial to maxillary deciduous canine and distal to mandibular deciduous canine.

26. In primary dentition, root calcification is completed 1-1.5 years post eruption. In permanent dentition root calcification is completed 2-3 years post eruption.

27. In Modelling, the child patient is encouraged to watch another person (Ideally a relaxed and reliable older sibling) to receive dental treatment.

Behaviour Shaping is a series of steps towards the ideal behaviour. In dental settings, the child patient can be rewarded for good behaviour at the end of each visit, for example by getting stickers or by using approving words and facial expressions.

28. Four benefits of nitrous oxide inhalation sedation:
    - Is suitable for treatment of patients with mild to moderate anxiety
    - Is preferred to general anaesthetic in orthodontic extractions
    - Acts as a weak analgesic
    - Has minimal effect on cardiovascular and respiratory function

29. Lignocaine 2% with 1:80,000 adrenaline is the first choice of anaesthesia and 1ml of solution is often enough to anaesthetise a primary tooth.

30. Four features associated with NAI:

- Pinch marks on the side of the ears
- Bilateral black eyes
- Bruise marks on the cheeks
- Fraenum tear in very young, non-ambulatory children

15 Radiography & Radiology: Questions

1. Name two regulations that apply to use of dental x-rays in UK?

2. Explain the differences in the roles of Radiation Protection Supervisor (RPS) and Radiation Protection Advisor (RPA).

3. Name six topics that should be included in Local Rules.

4. Explain the differences between "Absorbed Dose" and "Effective Dose".

5. What are the two main sources of radiation that can affect the dental staff?

6. What is the recommended thickness for aluminium filters in x-ray machines?

7. What is Focal Trough?

8. Name four shadows that can be mistaken for caries on a dental radiograph.

9. Name three advantages of Bitewing radiographs (BW) over Dental Panoramic Tomographs (DPT).

10. What are the two techniques used in taking Periapical radiographs?

11. What is a differential diagnosis for a round radiolucent lesion with a corticated margin at root apex which is smaller than 10mm in size?

12. Name two anatomical structures that appear radiolucent on dental radiographs.

13. Name three radiographs that can be used in periodontal assessment.

14. Name a differential diagnosis for "Ground Glass" appearance on a dental radiograph.

15. Describe radiographic features associated with Giant cell granuloma.

16. What is a differential diagnosis for a radiopaque round lesion associated with a resorbed root with a black margin which is continuous with the periodontal ligament (PDL)?

17. Name three advantages and three disadvantages of ultrasounds.

18. Name four indications for use of ultrasounds in dentistry.

19. Name two advantages and two disadvantages of Magnetic Resonance Imaging (MRI).

20. What are the three advantages and disadvantages of using Computed Tomography (CT) scans?

16 Radiography & Radiology: Answers

1. Two regulations for dental x-rays in UK:

Ionising Radiation Regulations 1999 (IRR99):

> This set of regulations is in place to reduce the risk of ionising radiations to dentists, dental nurses and other dental team members and to keep the risk as low as reasonably practicable (ALARP).

Ionising Radiations (Medical Exposures) Regulations 2000 (IR(ME)R):

> These regulations are in place to reduce patients' exposure to radiation.

2. Differences between RPS and RPA:

Radiation Protection Supervisor (RPS) is responsible for ensuring compliance with IRR99 in the area which is subject to Local

Rules. In dental practices, RPS is often the dentist or a senior member of the staff with adequate training.

Radiation Protection Advisor (RPA) provides advice to RPS regarding compliance with IRR99 to help protect staff and general public from ionising radiation. The RPA must hold a valid certificate from an organisation which is recognised by the Health and safety Executives (HSE).

3.   Six topics included in Local Rules:
- Name of the RPS
- Definition of the controlled area (1.5 meter from the x-ray tube, patient and the direct beam)
- Name and the training of the staff members who can takes radiographs
- Working instructions
- Details for dealing with equipment malfunction and accidental exposure
- Name and contact details for RPA

4. Absorbed Dose is the measure of radiation energy absorbed by unit mass of tissue. It is measured in Grays.

Effective Dose is the measure of potential long-term damage to the tissue.

5. Scattered radiation from patient and radiation leakage from tube head

6. Recommended thickness for aluminium filter is 2.5 mm

7. Focal Trough refers to the three-dimensional, horseshoe-shaped zone where images are sharp. The panoramic radiograph is composed of the anatomical structures within focal trough. Structures which fall in front or behind the focal trough can appear distorted. To obtain an accurate and clear image, patients must be positioned with their head carefully aligned in the focal trough.

8. Four shadows mistaken for caries:
  - Internal/external resorption
  - Toothbrush abrasion lesion
  - Restorations
  - Cervical burnout

9. Three advantages of BWs over DPTs:
- Bitewings provide higher resolution
- Bitewings allow more reproducible technique
- More accurate image with bitewings

10. Parallel technique and Bisected angle technique

11. Periapical granuloma

12. The two anatomical structures that appear radiolucent are:
- Mental foramen
- Nasopalatine foramen

13. Three radiographs used in periodontal assessments:
- Horizontal bitewing radiographs
- Periapical radiographs
- Dental panoramic tomographs

14. Fibrous dysplasia

15. Unilocular or multilocular radiolucent lesion with "Soap Bubble" appearance. The adjacent teeth may be resorbed or moved and it could also cause jaw expansion.

16. Benign cementoblastoma

17. Advantages of ultrasound:
- Non ionising
- Differentiates between soft tissues
- Quick

Disadvantages of ultrasound:
- Restricted to superficial structures
- Requires a skilled operator
- Presence of air or calcified areas can affect image quality

18. Four indications for use of ultrasound:
- Accessing lymph nodes
- Guidance for Fine Needle Aspiration
- Investigating salivary gland disease

19. Advantages of MRI:
- No ionising radiation is used
- Good at differentiating between different soft tissues

Disadvantages of MRI:

- Can't differentiate between teeth, bone and metallic objects
- Contraindicated in patients with cardiac pacemakers or during first semester of pregnancy

20. Advantages of CT scan:
- Good spatial resolution
- Shows good bone details
- Not contraindicated in patients with cardiac pacemakers

Disadvantages of CT scan:

- Uses ionising radiation
- Soft tissue differentiation is not as good as MRI
- Possible allergy to contrast medium

References

Gutmann, J.L. Dumsha, T.C. Lovdahl, P.E. (2006) *"Problem Solving in Endodontics"*, Elsevier Mosby, ISBN: 978-0-323-03182-0

Kidd, E.A.M. Smith, B.G.N. Pickard, H.M. (1993) *"Pickard's Manual of Operative Dentistry"*, Oxford Medical Publications, ISBN: 0-19-261808-3

Malet, J. Mora, F. Bouchard, P. (2012) *"Implant Dentistry at a Glance"*, John Wiley & Sons, ISBN: 978-1-4443-3744-0

Scully, C. Cawson, R.A. (2008) *"Medical Problems in Dentistry"*, Elsevier Churchill Livingstone, ISBN: 0-443-10145-0

Soames, J.V. Southam, J.C. (2003) *"Oral Pathology"*, Oxford University Press, ISBN: 0-19-262894-1

Van Beek, C.G. (1983) *"Dental Morphology"*, Wright PSG, ISBN: 0-7236-0666-8

Walmsley, A.D. Walsh, T.F. Lumley, P.J. Burke, F.J.T. Shortall, A.C. Hayes-Hall, R. Pretty, I.A. (2008)

"Restorative Dentistry", Churchill Livingstone, ISBN: 978-0-443-10246-2

Welbury, R.C. Duggal, S.M. Hosey, M. (2006) *"Peadiatric Dentistry"*, Oxford University Press, ISBN: 978-0-19-856583-3

Index